Praise f(

☞ Bill Burleigh has written a gem. His engaging personality, common sense and thinly disguised knowledge of endurance training all shine through. *Fitness Lite* is simple and humorous without sacrificing proper diet and valid training theory. Bill is living proof that fitness can be simple, easy and fun.

—FRANK SHORTER
First American Olympic Marathon Gold Medalist and top promoter of running as a popular sport

☞ This book is great! Bill uses his wit and knowledge to introduce people to fitness through running. His easy to understand, step-by-step approach to fitness will inspire all who read *Fitness Lite.*The beginning runner will find here all the motivation and information he needs.

—JOAN BENOIT SAMUELSON
Olympic Marathon Gold Medalist, 1984

☞ Bill Burleigh's *Fitness Lite* is beginner-friendly. It speaks your language, gives you a workable training plan, makes you smile. It's an appetizing first course in running.

—JOE HENDERSON
Author of *Fitness Running* and numerous other running books

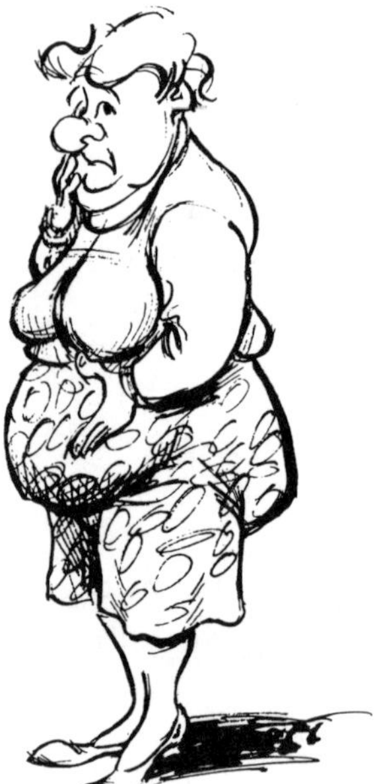

BEFORE
reading this book

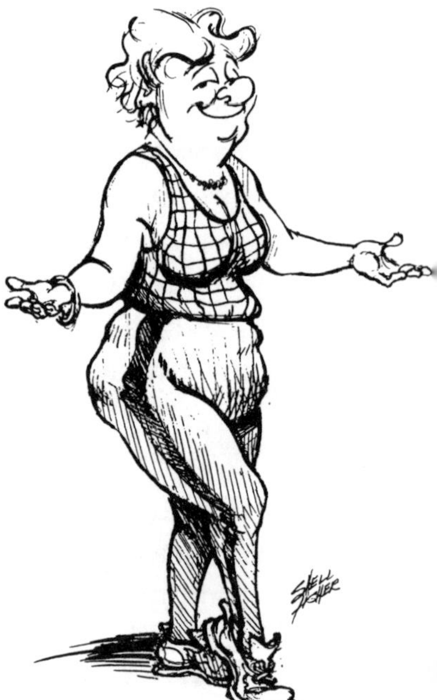

AFTER
reading this book

FITNESS Lite

A Guide For Those Who Have Never Taken Fitness Seriously

WILLIAM B. BURLEIGH

ILLUSTRATED BY SHELL FISHER

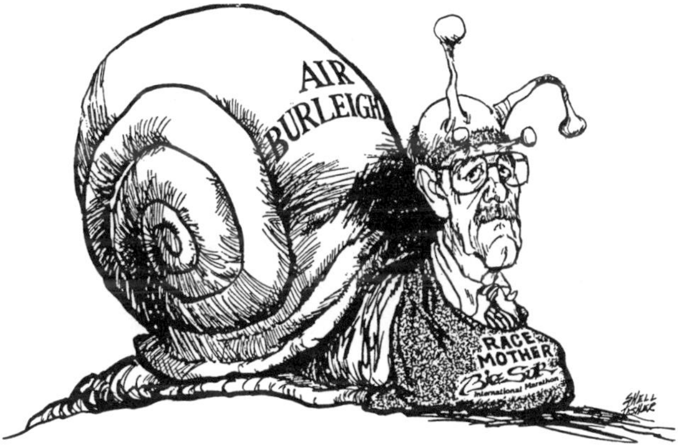

Capra Press

SANTA BARBARA

Printed in the United States of America

LIBRARY OF CONGRESS CATALOGING-IN-PUBLICATION DATA

Burleigh, William
Fitness lite : a guide for those who have never taken fitness seriously / William B. Burleigh : illustrated by Shell Fisher.
p. cm.
Based on a series of columns written for the Monterey County herald.
ISBN 0-88496-390-X (alk. paper)
1. Jogging. 2. Diet. 3. Physical Fitness. I. Title
GV494.B88 1994 CIP
813.7'172—dc20 94-45732

Art Director: Frank Goad
Printed by McNaughton & Gunn, Saline, MI

CAPRA PRESS
P.O. Box 2068, Santa Barbara, CA 93120

TABLE

Of What You Have To Look Forward To

PREFACE

I DON'T KNOW why this book has an introduction and a preface. I'm not even sure what a preface is, but this is probably as good a place as any to try and convince you that I know what I'm talking about. (With sentences like that one, I may have already lost you.)

My credentials are not impeccable, but adequate. I'm about half-fit and expect to stay that way indefinitely. My weight fluctuates, from real tight pants at the waist to semi-tight pants, and I'm generally about ten pounds overweight. When I started running I was easily 30-40 pounds overweight.

I began a very modest program of running about 19 years ago. During that time I've run hundreds of foot-races, mostly 3, 5 and 6.2 milers, plus three 26.2 mile marathons.

"Races," in my case, is a misnomer. I run so slowly that no one would call it racing. I'm known in running circles as Ice Flow Burleigh—you can't get any slower than a glacier. (Maybe you can—I was recently called Continental Drift Burleigh.) But I eventually finish the distance, nevertheless.

I was the founder and director of a successful 10 K (6.2 mile) race in Big Sur, California, for four years. I then started the Big Sur Marathon, currently in its tenth year and ranked among the top 20 marathons in the country: 7,000 participants and a $400,000. budget. Both events have flourished because, in part, we don't take the sport too seriously, and encourage our participants to run for pleasure rather than athletic achievement.

I'm not a nutritionist, but my wife has read all the books and taken all the courses, and I have learned the subject by osmosis. I don't always eat properly, but I know how it's done. You know, do what I say, not what I do. I'm good at quoting authorities. All the chapters in this book have been approved for accuracy by orthopedic surgeons, exercise physiologists, registered dieticians, and podiatrists, whichever was appropriate.

In other words, you can believe what you read.

This book is based on a series of columns I wrote for the daily newspaper in my community, the *Monterey County Herald*. Many readers (2) suggested that I write a book.

In my other life I am a judge, which may or may not have some significance.

A More Important Than Usual
INTRODUCTION

IF YOU DON'T read this introduction you have wasted your $9.95. This may be the most important part of the whole book: What I am trying to do.

I'm not writing this just for the people who want to take care of themselves, who exercise occasionally, who "eat their vegetables." I'm writing this also for the couch potato, the overweight, dissipated, lethargic, unhealthy, normal human being. What some call the Road Slug.

If you read this book, and do what I tell you, you may still be overweight, dissipated, lethargic and unhealthy, but only about half as much as you used to be. You will definitely feel better.

How does this amazing semi-transformation take place? Quite easily, believe it or not. Because what this book seeks to do is make you feel better than you do now, and live longer, without working too hard.

Most fitness advice is hard to take—too much sweat, too much hunger, too much suffering.

This book is different. The amount of time, money and effort demanded is minimal. You can still eat what you want most of the time, watch all the TV you can handle, and sleep 'til noon on weekends.

The total cost of this program is about a dollar or two a week. If you can afford this book, you can afford the cost of semi-fitness. Actually, if you adopt some of my suggestions on food, you'll end up saving more money than you spend.

The amount of time you spend on this program is only about an hour or two a week. I don't even demand much of you intellectually. There are 16 chapters of a few pages each. All you have to do is set aside a few minutes to read a chapter each week for four months, and follow the directions.

My point is that anyone, no matter what age, physical condition, weight, economic status or social demands, can complete this program with very little effort. If you are not physically disabled, this book is for you.

Although the program is built around training for a 5K (3.1 mile) footrace, this is not a running book; it is, rather, a gentle change-in-lifestyle book.

And here's the good part: if you follow this simple program, I absolutely guarantee that 16 weeks from now you will feel better than you do today. And you'll probably look better. And maybe live longer, but even if you don't, you'll feel better while you're alive.

Go for it!

William B. Burleigh
Carmel, California
August 7, 1994

WEEK ONE

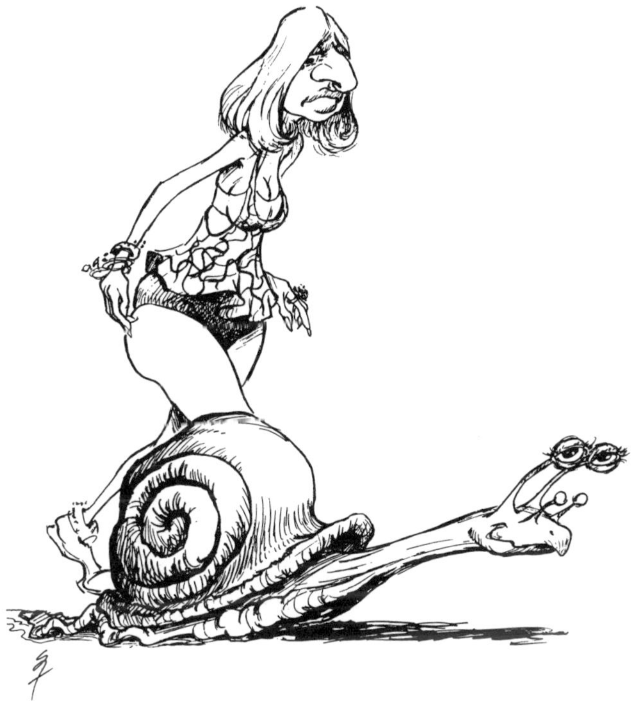

The First Steps to Semi-fitness Are, Well, a Shuffle

IF YOU DIDN'T read the introduction to this book, go back and do so. If you don't, the book will self-destruct.

Alright, now you're ready to get started. Get off the couch, open the yellow pages and find the name of the closest running store/sport shop. We're starting at the bottom: your feet.

This will be your single biggest, and perhaps only, expense. You need a good pair of running shoes. Whatever they cost, you will probably make up the cost with future dietary changes.

This is about the only thing in this book that I take seriously, and insist that you do as well. You have to get good quality, light-weight, name-brand running shoes. Not tennies, sneakers or cross-trainers. I want you in comfortable shoes that only weigh a few ounces.

Don't go to a discount store and buy shoes on sale; you could be getting seconds that may be flawed, and cheap shoes will defeat the whole program. Get name brands only: Asics, New Balance, Nike, Reebok, Etonic, Mizuno, Brooks, Saucony, Avia, Adidas, Diadora or Turntec. If the shoes are not on this list, don't buy them.

Unfortunately, name is not enough. Different feet need different kinds of shoes. When I began running, I didn't know the importance of a good fit. Over time I had to buy and wear three different brands before I found the perfect shoe. The first two I tried left me with sore knees or bruised heels. A responsible running store will help you get the right fit, and stand behind their advice.

If you pay less than $60, you're taking a risk on quality and taking the risk of injury. You want to end up with the comfort and weight of slippers.

Next, ask the sales clerk at the running store for a copy of the schedule of local footraces. The major running magazines, *Runner's World* and *Running Times* are primarily for experienced runners and only list races one month in advance. You need the newsprint, tabloid style booklet that lists races for most of the year.

Now, pick out a 5K (3.1 mile) race four months from now. A full page ad would probably be a good bet. You may have to travel 20-40 miles for a good 5K. If you're having trouble finding one, ask the sales clerk or some good local runners.

You now are ready! You have good shoes and a goal: to run a 5K footrace 16 weeks from now. Don't be intimidated; you can do it.

Anyone who isn't disabled can run 3.1 miles without stopping or walking. All it takes is a little training, a little conditioning. I'm going to tell you how to do that with the least amount of pain and suffering.

I'm not going to make your life miserable, or demand more than you can handle. There will be some mild discomfort, primarily the first few weeks, but the rewards will exceed the effort.

☆

Your training starts now. Put on your new shoes, go down to the local school track, and jog a little. Walk for 50 yards or so, then trot for 50-60 feet. Yes, feet, not yards. Then walk for awhile. You should be able to do one lap around the track (¼ mile) in five minutes.

Depending on how much time you have, try this two to five times a week, for about 10 minutes each time. Don't push, don't run hard or fast, and don't strain.

The biggest mistake beginning runners make is actually running. Don't do it. It's discouraging, uncomfortable and even painful. What you want during these first few weeks is a shuffle! Your body isn't ready for running, and you could injure yourself.

☆

Get out there and shuffle. Until next week, Happy Feet!

WEEK TWO

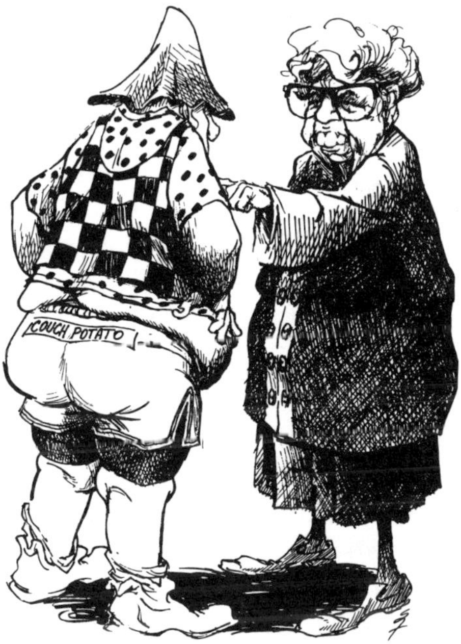

If you leave the house dressed like that, I'm changing the locks.

Training One Step Beyond Going to the Refrigerator

WHEN I LEFT YOU last week, I had you in good quality, lightweight, $60 running shoes, shuffling a little bit on the high school track. You are reluctantly approaching a major change in your lifestyle.

A couple more points in preparation before I get you started. One: if you are an over-40 non-athlete, and you have never put physical stress on your heart, you should get your doctor's approval before starting to train. If you have a history of heart disease in your family, you should also consider getting a treadmill stress test. Actually, you would enjoy comparing your treadmill results now with your results after four months. Big ego trip.

Even if you yourself have had heart problems, even a heart attack, your cardiologist will probably give you a gold star for getting involved with exercise and fitness, even semi-fitness.

Since you are beginning to change your lifestyle, it would be nice to have some empirical proof of your improved fitness. So I want you to get a professional to give you your cholesterol (good and bad), lipids, blood pressure and pulse. You'll be amazed at the changes, good changes, you will see in the next three months. There's a chart at the end of this book; fill in the left column as soon as you get your test results.

Secondly, a brief word about clothing. For the level of training that you are going to be doing, any old clothing is okay. Any kind of shorts or pants, a raggedy old T-shirt and wind breaker, and when it's cold, some cotton garden gloves. The only thing of importance is comfort.

I'm going to hold your hand for the next four months and you are going to gently and quietly learn to run 3.1 miles, without stopping. Or hurting.

My program is a modest one, designed to improve fitness and general health. You can still OD on ice cream occasionally, sleep in 'til noon on weekends, watch all the football, baseball, soap operas and game shows on

TV, take naps at will, and eat all the pretzels you want.

But you will eventually feel subtle changes. Your weight may not drop too much, but the circumference of some of your body parts will, as they slowly change from fat to muscle.

Are you ready to get started?

At least mentally?

Here goes. Let's get physical.

Some runners like to stretch muscles, particularly in the legs, before running, but at your starting speed and effort, you probably don't need to. (That is a grammatically permissible dangling participle.)

If you do choose to stretch, do it S-L-O-W-L-Y. Stand on the edge of the curb and work your calves, by raising and lowering yourself on the balls of your feet. You can feel your calves stretch. Next, pick up a foot and gently pull it up behind you. Finally, lean into a wall, fence or car, with one leg straight out, and gently stretch your hamstrings. Ten minutes of this is more than enough.

When you start running, run as slowly as you can, then cut your speed in half. Walk around corners if you aren't on the track. Avoid hills. The school track is boring, but it has the virtues of being flat, a measured distance (almost always one-fourth mile), and no traffic.

I want you on a track (or if that's not convenient, on a flat, measured, no-traffic area) for a few weeks. It's the perfect starting place. Assuming it is a track for a public school, it is paid for by your taxes. You can't interfere with the track team, but you can use the track while the football team is practicing.

To reduce the boredom, you can get an AM-FM cassette player for under $40, or a headset, and listen to your favorite cassettes or switch it to radio for news, sports, weather, talk shows or your favorite FM station.

I have to repeat: the biggest mistake beginning runners make is running. When I say I want you to run, I don't mean sprint. When you are starting out, run as slow as you can, then run a little bit slower.

For the first couple weeks, don't run for more than two minutes without walking, and don't total more than ten minutes. Even that amount of exercise will be uncomfortable and unpleasant. But hang in there. If you can force yourself to keep at it for a few months, it gets easier and easier. There's even a good chance that you will come to enjoy it and start a lifetime of feeling better.

The distance you cover is not important. I just want you to remain vertical and in motion for the first couple of weeks of training. Speed is not relevant. Actually, maybe it is: the slower, the better.

Remember: a slow jog, indeed a shuffle, on a school track, for not more than two minutes, then walk. After about 9-10 minutes, go home and have a soda or a beer. Do this three times a week.

☆

Next week I will tell you how to strengthen the most important muscle in your body. Until then, Happy Feet!

WEEK THREE

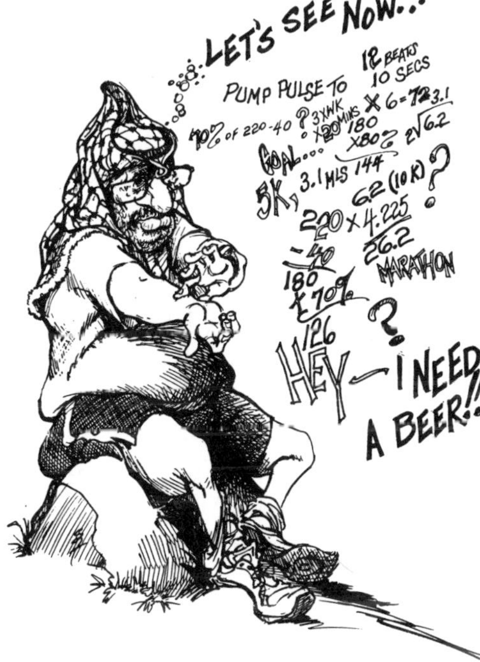
LET'S SEE NOW...
PUMP PULSE TO
12 BEATS 10 SECS
GOAL...
MARATHON
HEY—I NEED A BEER!!

Building Up the Most Important Muscle in your Body

HEREWITH MORE fitness advice for those who are satisfied with being semi-fit; those who want to be able to finish the 5K footrace fourteen weeks from now.

Last week I left you in a slow shuffle and walk around your school track, for about 10 minutes at a time, three times a week.

This week, as promised, I am going to get you into a little muscle work; more specifically, that all-important muscle called your heart. Since this book is directed primarily toward the sedentary person of any age, I will assume that you have the heart of a normal sedentary person. (And that your doctor approves of this training.)

First, while you're sitting there reading this, touch the side of your throat, or your wrist below your thumb, and take your pulse rate. Count the number of beats in 10 seconds and multiply by six. You are probably about 70-75 beats per minute, the same rate I had when I started running.

My present resting pulse is about 50-55, which is normal for anyone who gets regular aerobic exercise.

So what's my point? It's this: your heart has the responsibility of getting your blood, with oxygen and all sorts of other good things, throughout your body. A stronger heart is a better heart.

For about half an hour, or 45 minutes, three to five times a week, my pulse rate is about 130-150, because I am running. That "aerobic" exercise strengthens my heart. The rest of the day my heart thumps along slowly. (Unless my daughter dented the car again, or the dog ate my wallet.)

During a normal day, your heart will beat almost 30,000 times more than mine—unnecessarily. If your heart only has so many beats built into it, it can only take so much activity, like a car. You are going to wear out your heart faster than me.

Your heart is like your bicep or your calf; the more you exercise it, the bigger and stronger it gets.

You can get your pulse rate down to the low 50s by a regular program of running. That's the bad news. The good news is that all you have to do is 20 minutes of running, three times a week.

Remember Dr. Kenneth Cooper's studies for the Air Force in the early 70s? He concluded, and it is still the accepted authority, that all you need to do for a healthy heart is 20 minutes of aerobic exercise three times a week.

(There was a recent highly publicized report that walking is as effective for improving health as running; the report is controversial and not accepted by all authorities.)

Dr. Cooper said that if you run more than twenty minutes, three times a week, you are doing it for reasons other than health. Believe it or not, and it's hard to even conceive of this when you are starting to run, there's a good chance you will run a lot, simply because you enjoy it and it feels good. Also, if you advance to the stage of running longer distances, and actually want to join your friends in a race, or even compete, you will run to prepare for the race.

Then again, I must concede that running isn't for everyone. My wife and I started running at the same time; I got hooked and she didn't. She now walks, including eight marathons, but she says she envies the benefits I get from running. I hope that after this four month program you are hooked, but don't feel bad if you aren't. At least you gave it your best shot, and found it wanting.

You are now ready for the most difficult part of your training: You need to work your way up to an elevated pulse rate for 20 minutes continuously, three times a week. You determine your optimum pulse rate by subtracting your age from 220, then taking 70 percent of that (80 percent for advanced runners). For example, a 40 year old beginning runner would try to maintain a pulse rate of about 126 (220-40 = 180, 70% of 180 is 126), and 144 pulse rate for experienced runners.

I have always had a hard time taking my pulse, either resting or during a run. I'm seldom confident that my count is accurate.

If you have the same problem, don't despair. Nice people in some laboratory have created a little device called a pulse monitor. It straps on your chest, under your breasts, and transmits your pulse to a wrist watch receiver. All you need to do is check your watch periodically to see if you are maintaining a rate high enough to get aerobic benefits and strengthen your heart. Or, by the same token, to see if you are pushing too hard, risking injury.

I run very slowly, about 9-11 minutes per mile, depending on how I feel, and I find that my pulse rate, as registered on the pulse monitor, is just about where it should be.

You can borrow or rent a monitor at your local running store, track club, running club, high school or college. Or, if you choose, you can purchase a good quality monitor for about $150. Check the ads in the running magazines.

It will take you a few weeks to work yourself up to your optimum pulse rate for 20 minutes, and it might be the most unpleasant and uncomfortable physical thing you have ever done. Just remember this: it gets easier and easier as time goes by. Your body feels heavy and sluggish now. In another 14 weeks you will float.

And if you are a typical runner, you will reach a point where you look forward to your run. It's a pleasant, sensual experience (even, upon occasion, exhilarating!), and you will run more than necessary, simply because it feels good.

And, while you are getting your pulse rate up, you are also preparing your body for a 3.1 mile run, the 5K you have chosen as your goal.

(This chapter has been approved by a medical doctor with a speciality in internal medicine/cardio-pulmonary.)

☆

Next week I am going to give you a short course on fuel. It's all part of this fitness business. In the meantime, Happy Feet! And eat your oranges.

WEEK FOUR

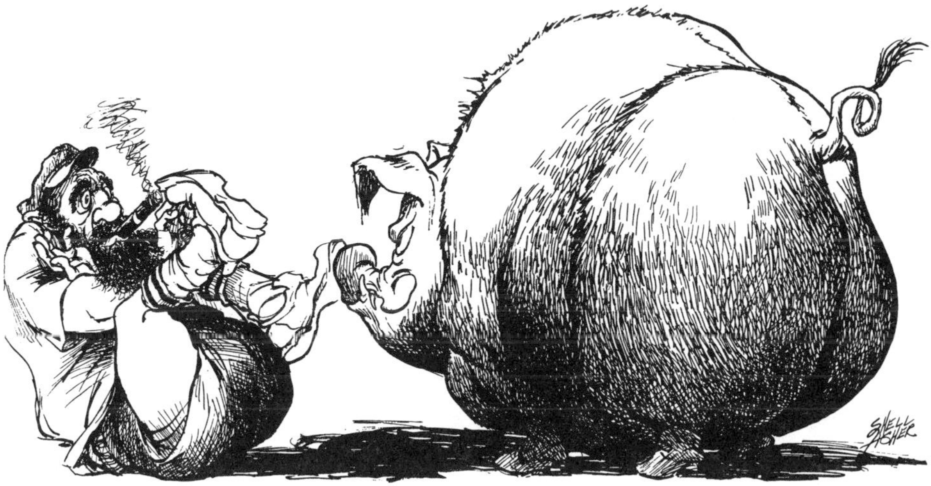

Fuels for the Body; Fuels that Burn Clean and Fuels that Burn Dirty

WELCOME BACK to the fitness book that doesn't take fitness too seriously. It's advice for those who want to improve their health enough to run a 3.1 mile footrace, without too much suffering.

When we left you last week, you were starting the

toughest part of your program—getting your pulse rate up to 120-150 beats per minute (depending on your age and condition), for 20 minutes at a time, three times a week. You probably haven't reached that goal yet—it often takes many weeks—but hang in there. When you reach that level, your fitness program is essentially down hill from there—a nice direction for runners.

This week we are introducing you to the best fuels for your body—but we are going to be realistic about it. Remember the book a couple of years ago, *Eat to Win?* Well, this chapter can be called "Eat to come in 842nd out of 1,000." But finish the distance, nevertheless.

Your body needs all kinds of stuff to keep going—including the much maligned fats and sugars. The key is in the proportion of your food intake that is attributable to fat and sugar.

There are lots of books that can tell you how many calories you need to maintain good health in relation to your weight and age. For instance, two good choices are Covert Bailey's *Fit or Fat*, or Nancy Clark's *Sports Nutrition Guide-book*. For our purposes, let's take a healthy, 150 pound person that needs about 2,000 calories a day.

Those calories can be in the form of protein (meats, cheeses, some vegetables), carbohydrates (pasta, breads, potatoes, rice), and fats (oils, butters, meat fats). This week we'll look at fats.

Ideally, you shouldn't have more than 600-700 calories a day in fat, and certainly no more than 30% of your total calorie intake.

Unfortunately, that's not a lot of fat, because fats are high in calories. One tablespoon of olive oil is 130 calories, almost a fourth of your recommended intake. So choose your fats carefully.

And always choose fats that are low in saturated fats. Animal fats (marbled red meat, cheeses, whole milk) are generally bad fats.

Happily, there are some terrific fat substitutes that trick you into thinking you are eating the real thing. Non-fat sour cream is the latest addition, and light margarine, non-dairy frozen desserts and low-fat cheese make life in the fat lane almost bearable.

You can have waffles with whipped cream for breakfast, chili for lunch, and for dinner you can splurge on refried beans smothered in cheese, tuna salad with mayonnaise, chocolate chip loaf and pound cake à la mode—and take in hardly any fat! It's a miracle! (See "Prevention Magazine," October, 1991.)

Here's a technique we have used in our family for many years, with fairly good success: We simply don't buy animal fats at the market: red meat, (unless it's lean—really lean), butter, bacon, ice cream, most cheeses. Our diet at home is full of pastas, breads, chicken, fish, salads, fruits, vegetables—seasoned with mostly non-fat sauces, such as yogurt or sour cream, and non-cholesterol oils. Our milk is non-fat, and we eat light cheeses.

You will be pleasantly surprised at the total of your bill at the check-out stand in the super market. Foods that you want to avoid—real ice cream, pork, potato chips, cookies and crackers—are not only high in fat, but high in cost. It has been years since we've bought a roast or T-bone at the store, and our food bills show it.

On the other hand, food that you need for good health—veggies, salads, fruit, pastas, potatoes—are inexpensive. You could live forever, in good health, on a diet of potatoes, broccoli, bananas and non-fat milk. Unless you died of boredom in the third month.

By behaving ourselves at home, we can rationalize eating bad foods away from home—the office picnic, dinner with friends, Monday Night Football hot dogs with the guys, neighborhood parties, etc.

If I have spent a week eating steamed vegetables, pastas, salads and fruit, I can easily justify dinner with the boss on Friday night, or a bacon omelette brunch Sunday morning. After a few weeks of careful eating, you can rationalize a multitude of sins.

We do cheat at home, but it's informed, intelligent cheating. We look at the nutrition label and check to see the proportion of fat to calories, and if it is over 30 percent, we try to avoid it.

For instance, if you look at the label on a box of Hi Ho Crackers, you'll see that for every 80 calories, there are 5 grams of fat. Each gram of fat is nine calories; (remember, your goal with fats, good or bad, is to keep them below 30 percent of your total food calorie intake.) That's almost 60% percent fat—and its a bad fat, too, saturated. You could go to jail for eating too many crackers.

On the other hand, Poppers Potato Chips (air popped,

then baked, not fried) have one half a gram of fat for every 50 calories—4½ calories, or less than 10% fat. That's a good snack. But remember, if you're weight conscious, they are still calories and will still add pounds to the body. Moderation, okay?

So much for fat. Next week we talk about the main power source for your body, the stamina fuel for your thrice weekly 20 minute runs. Until then, Happy Feet! And eat your veggies.

☆

(The advice on this chapter has been approved by registered nutritionists at the Community Hospital of the Monterey Peninsula, Carmel, California.)

WEEK FIVE

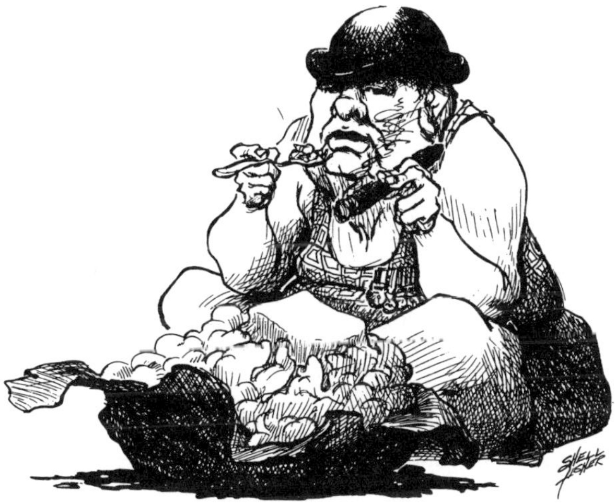

Do I Really Have to Eat that Fettucini Alfredo with Sour Cream and Cheese Sauce?

WE ARE STARTING our fifth week of training for the 5K (3.1 mile) run, 11 weeks down the road. So to speak.

You are struggling to keep your pulse rate around 130-150 beats per minute, three times a week, while slowly jogging around the local high school track for 20 minutes.

This is the low point of your fitness plan because you haven't yet trained your body to store glycogen and pump oxygen efficiently to your muscles. That will come with time—just keep at it.

Last week we discussed how to limit your fat intake. This week we give you the most remarkable fuel source you put into your body: carbohydrates.

We use the word "remarkable" because you can actually feel the effect on your stamina and endurance when you eat pasta before a long distance run. It seems like a miracle.

Exercise physiologists and nutritionists like to refer to this fuel as glycogen. It's easier to use the common name: carbohydrates.

Remember when, 30 years ago, football teams fed their athletes thick steaks before a game for energy and power? No more; go to a football training table and check the plates of lasagna, fettuccini, potatoes and bread, and some fruits. There's a good reason for this change in diet for athletes: carbohydrates are the single greatest source of energy for your muscles.

It would be nice if you could just eat a few potatoes and then use that fuel to run 10 miles. Unfortunately, you have to train your muscles to accept and store the glycogen, then parcel it out as needed. The only way this can be done is to run long distances. Actually, any repetitive, sustained use of muscle, such as swimming, or walking, will increase storage capacity, but for our purposes in preparing for the 5K, running is best. As your level of fitness slowly improves, you will be able to run longer and longer distances without stopping and without too much suffering. You can easily illustrate the value of carbohydrates by eating a vegetable dinner, then go for a five-mile run the next day. Tough. Then eat a pasta dinner and do the same run. Piece of cake.

A good pre-endurance event meal could be: 1 ½ cups of egg noodles (300 calories); 1 cup non-fat yogurt sauce with Romano cheese (180); one 7 oz. baked potato (220) with 2 tablespoons non-fat sour cream (50); 1 cup steamed broccoli and carrots (50) with soy sauce (20); 1 medium banana (100) lettuce and tomato with non-fat dressing (about 100). That's a healthy and tasty 1,000 plus calorie dinner.

It's interesting how science changes our perceptions of things. Older readers will remember that about 20 years ago the meal described above would be a no-no. Too fattening. Too much "starch" as they used to call it. Anyone that wanted to control their weight tried to avoid breads and potatoes and rice. No more. As you will see in later chapters, these foods are not only permitted in a weight loss program, but encouraged because of their value in giving us energy.

I hope scientific knowledge eventually reaches the point of discovering that chocolate is a critical element of a balanced diet.

If you question the importance of carbohydrates and endurance, look at the entry form for any major marathon. They all offer a carbo party the night before the 26.2 mile race.

I am going to urge you to load up on spaghetti, bread, potatoes, fruit, etc., before your 5K run. It will make a difference. (Mainly because you will weigh 300 pounds and you won't be able to move. Just kidding; more on weight control later.)

☆

Keep putting one foot in front of the other. You will eventually get there. Happy Feet! And eat your carrots.

WEEK SIX

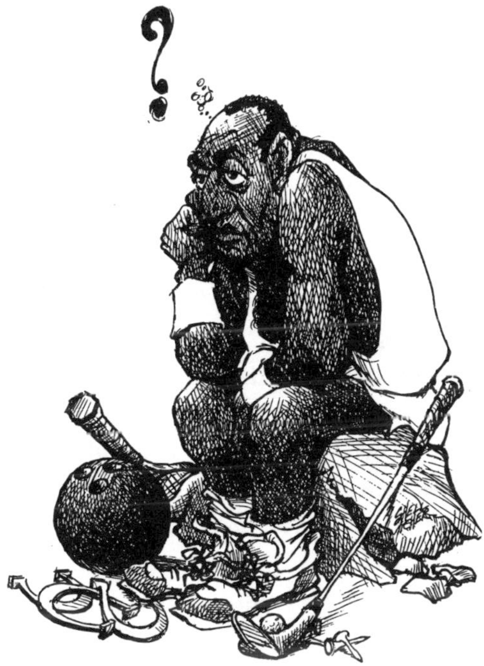

Running will Make You Rich and Famous. Well . . .

WHY RUN?

Indeed, that's a good question. Why should a person risk injury to his or her knees, ankles, feet or hips by the incessant pounding you get with road running? Why not get your exercise, your good health, your fitness, from activities that do less damage?

Wouldn't you be better off swimming, cycling, or playing tennis, golf or racquetball?

The answer, I submit, is no. For overall satisfaction, running is the best of all activities. Here's why:

1. *Aerobic benefits.* You need at least 20 minutes of increased pulse rate, three times a week, for a strong, healthy heart, reduced cholesterol, lowered blood pressure, stronger bones, etc. That's easy with running, but impossible with golf and downhill skiing, and not likely with tennis, walking or resistance training. Only swimming provides the same benefits aerobically, but it's so ... wet. Singles tennis gets your pulse rate up, but it isn't sustained for 20 minutes. Just little bursts.

2. *Anybody can do it.* You don't have to be an athlete to run. You don't have to have hand-eye coordination or muscles, a good body or a competitive instinct.

I have the athletic skills and coordination of an aged rhinoceros, but I still get immense pleasure from an hour of putting one foot in front of the other. My reflexes are too slow for tennis. I tried golf for years and seldom broke 100. And it was no pleasure.

The same benefits come with cycling, and probably swimming, but you need skill for tennis, golf or skiing.

3. *Running is probably the least expensive of all aerobic activities.* All you need is a pair of good quality, lightweight running shoes. With normal wear and tear, you can run all you want for about a dollar a week.

Compare that to the cost of a bicycle, ski lift tickets, golf club memberships or swimming privileges. Or stables, if you are into polo.

Only walking can compare in cost and it doesn't give you the same aerobic benefits, and walking takes about twice as long to get the same calorie burn.

4. *There's very little fuss involved in running.* You don't need to make arrangements for meeting others, as in golf, skiing or tennis. You don't need another human being as a partner. A lot of runners enjoy the escape of running, a chance to be alone with yourself, with no obligations or social intercourse. A time to think, plan, scheme.

It's just as well that it can be done alone: I run so slowly that I wouldn't be able to find anyone to run with me. Well, I take that back. My golden retriever runs with me. But he's on a leash.

5. *No other non-aerobic activity releases that magic chemical in your brain called endorphin.* Everyone has heard of the "runner's high," that feeling of elation, well-being, riding on top of the world, that happens occasionally with the long-distance runner.

Have you ever heard of a golf high?

I must reluctantly admit that a workout on one of those cross-country ski machines gives you aerobic benefits without damage to your joints. These machines, however, have led to numerous verified deaths by boredom.

☆

Finally, I concede that running isn't for everyone. I know several people, including my wife, that gave it a good try and found it wanting. She turned to walking, a legitimate and healthy activity, and we respect each other's choices.

It's hard for me to acknowledge that you don't really need vigorous aerobic exercise to be fit.

Increasing your pulse rate for 20 minutes, three times a week, is good for you, and it does make a stronger heart, but if you take three 10-minute walks every day you will probably accomplish about the same results.

That's the conclusion of the Center of Science in the Public Interest, as reported in their popular magazine, *Nutrition Action*, December, 1993.

This is one of my favorite periodicals, and it has given the public hard-hitting, non-political fitness information for years.

"Just a half hour a day of moderate exercise like walking, dancing, bicycling or swimming can lower your risk of dying almost as much as a regimen of vigorous exercise. And it doesn't have to be 30 minutes in a row." The cover story then prints interviews with seven leading researchers. Steven N. Blair, Director of Epidemiology at the Institute for Aerobics Research, Dallas: A moderate amount of exercise increases HDL, the good cholesterol, he says, and lowers your blood pressure, makes you less likely to gain weight, increases insulin sensitivity in the muscles, and lowers the risk of forming blood clots.

"The key thing is to get up and get moving and not

worry about intensity. It's the total energy spent in physical activity that's most important." says Blair.

This is good stuff I'm passing on to you, so pay attention. If you accept what Blair and many others say, it cuts down on your excuses for not exercising.

I mean, how can you say you didn't have time to walk around the block a few times? And you certainly aren't risking injury by just walking.

If you can't bring yourself to get off the couch, keep this statement from the American College of Sports Medicine in mind: "A staggering quarter of a million deaths each year can be attributed to physical inactivity." This same statistic is given by the Center for Disease Control and the President's Council on Physical Fitness.

☆

I am compelled, however, to put in a plea for activity in any form. Although I think running is pleasurable, anything that makes you move is good for you.

I know there are many who feel that your ticket has already been punched, that fate has picked your date for you. Perhaps, but why not enjoy the trip? It is an absolute truth that you simply feel better after you exercise.

☆

Until next week, Happy Feet! And eat your cauliflower.

WEEK SEVEN

It says here, if it's a dull ache, just keep running.

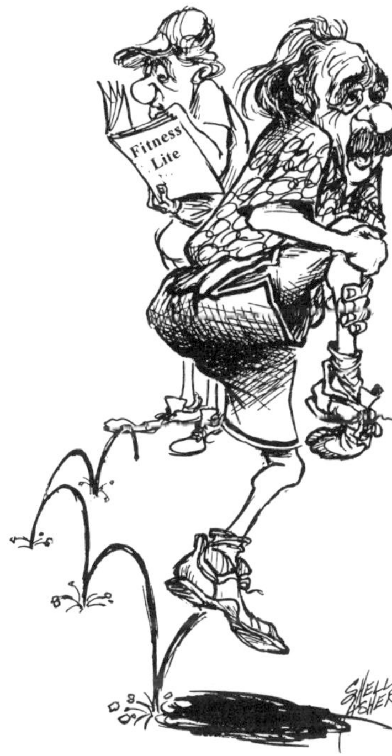

It Only Hurts When I Cry

FOR THOSE SEEKING a moderately realistic level of fitness, welcome to the seventh week of almost tolerable fitness advice. For those turning out the light, good night; rest well.

Thus far, we have you slowly grinding out a few miles

a week, keeping your pulse rate up, eating properly and moving into a new lifestyle.

This week we want to get you up to date on pain and injury. This is not medical advice; rather, we just want to keep you out of trouble with your body during your training for the 5K.

Ideally this information will be useless; you will become fit without mishap. Realistically, if you train properly, you will have some minor pain and perhaps some injury.

A general rule for pain is this: if it is a dull ache, it will probably go away as you run. If it's a sharp pain, stop. If it persists, see your doctor.

All kinds of things happen inside your body when you run—mostly good, some bad. We'll talk about the good things some other week, but for now let's consider the less-than-pleasant.

Besides overall exhaustion, the most common discomfort you are likely to experience is the "side-stitch". It's a bothersome pain in the side of your stomach, caused by a muscle strain or spasm. It's generally an annoyance to beginning runners, and as you become aerobically healthy, it will become a thing of the past. I haven't had a side-stitch for about 20 years.

In the meantime, when it hits, you can almost always eliminate it by stopping and pressing your fingers against the spot that hurts; that will dissipate the spasm and almost always stop the pain. (One school of thought attributes the pain to a gas bubble in the intestines; no matter, pressure usually relieves it.)

The next most common pain you will find is the heel bruise. But if you followed our advice in the first chapter and bought good quality running shoes, you might avoid this annoyance.

If you still experience the heel pain, like I did, switch brands of shoes until you get one that cures the problem. If that doesn't work, see a podiatrist or an orthopedist. Don't let it keep you from getting fit.

Another common pain (usually due to inadequate water, training or diet) is cramping. As you become more fit and learn to eat and drink properly, cramping will not likely bother you. Cramping is caused by lack of water, potassium, calcium, salt and/or magnesium, or inadequate stretching before exercise. Once the cramp begins, though, stretch the muscle until it goes away.

For instance, you can eliminate a cramp in the arch of your foot by curling your toes up and stretching out the muscles in your arch. If it's your calf, turn your whole foot up and pull out the calf muscle. This tip is worth the price of this book; I wish someone had told me about this simple cure a few decades ago—it would have saved a lot of discomfort—including cramps that go ouch in the night.

If your leg or ankle or foot hurts and you can't figure out where, press around until you hit a tender spot. If it's around a joint, it's probably tendinitis—soft tissue rheumatism. Ibuprofen (Advil, Motrin, etc.) ice or heat and rest might be enough to cure it in a few days. If not, see your doctor.

A brochure from American Running and Fitness Association describes other common injuries, and their remedies:

A common knee injury is patella (knee-cap)-femoral (bone behind the kneecap) compression syndrome. (Chrondomalacia patella. Really interesting, right?) This pain happens when the knee cap slams into the femur.

It is often caused by excessive pronation, or muscle weakness around the knee. Rest and icing should temporarily reduce pain. Orthotics may reduce further flare-ups. Try strengthening your quadriceps with resistance work (weight or machines) to cut back on the pain.

Another common cause of knee pain is illotibial band syndrome (ITBS), which causes pain on the outside of the knee. The start of the pain is slow and occurs after running a certain distance.

The major causes of ITBS are excessive internal rotation of the leg and pronation of the subtalar joint. Both cause the ITB to be stretched over a bony priminence of the femur (the bone in your thigh), which leads to irritation and later, pain. Treatment includes rest, icing, eliminating over-pronation, and stretching the ITB.

Is this fun reading or what? You could be reading *Calvin and Hobbes* at this very moment.

The last injury I want to talk about is brain strain. It commonly occurs when reading really dull books and is generally accompanied by drowsiness and, occasionally, headache.

Treatment includes rest, icing—preferably after removal from the cranium—and anti-inflammatories. Some runners have obtained relief from a '91 Merlot.

The last couple paragraphs were tossed in to see if you are awake. If you are still reading this, you have an abnormal and suspicious interest in pain.

Just a final serious note: don't give up your active lifestyle because it occasionally hurts. I have friends who were active runners, but have turned into road slugs because of pain and the fear of more injury. If you can't run, walk. If you can't walk, bike. If you can't bike, swim.

The benefits you get from exercise, mentally, physically and emotionally, far exceed most of the injuries you suffer from running or other activities. Hang in there.

Finally, keep in mind that a certain amount of pain and discomfort is inevitable if you are active. Just remember that you are strengthening your heart, making your bones harder, lowering your cholesterol, blood pressure and pulse rate and increasing your longevity. And, of most importance, you are improving your sense of well-being and self-esteem. You're worth it.

(The advice in this chapter has been approved by a physician with a specialty in orthopedics.)

☆

Keep on shuffling and trudging around that track. This is the low point of your training, the time you might get discouraged. So, next week is inspiration time. Until then, Happy Feet! And eat your potatoes!

WEEK EIGHT

Oh great spirit of runners, my endorphins didn't kick in, so how 'bout you finishing my run today?

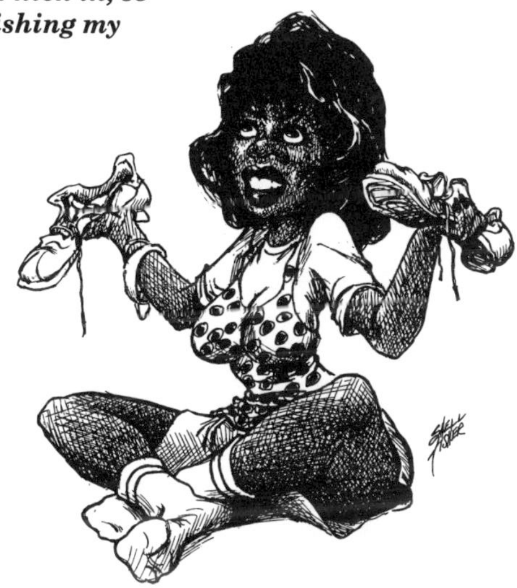

If You Can Fog a Mirror, You Can Be an Athlete

YOU HAVE BEEN struggling along now for seven weeks, and things may be getting grim. You are still in the most difficult stage of your training for the 5K, and sometimes it gets discouraging. Perhaps it's time for a little inspiration.

We want to show you that anyone without a physical disability can run 3.1 miles. And attain at least moderate fitness.

I am living proof that any human who can fog a mirror can run a marathon. If I can do that, I assure you that if your body is warm to the touch, you can run several miles without effort.

When I turned 40, I didn't like how I felt or what I saw in the mirror. I was overweight, smoking heavily, often tired and probably drinking more than I should. My joints hurt, my stomach ached and, most importantly, my head wasn't in good shape.

Someone said you can turn your life around by jogging, so I thought I would at least try it for a few months. The first few weeks were awful. I couldn't jog 50 yards without gasping. Everything hurt. It was weeks before I could make it around the high school track.

Then after about three months, I had my first good run. That magic chemical in the brain they call endorphin kicked in, and I enjoyed my first "runner's high", a feeling of elation and well-being. It lasted for hours and hours.

And now, after 18 years of regular running, I'm still overweight, smoking, drinking too much (. . . no, no, no— just funning). I am still somewhat overweight, but I eat a lot and I hate to think what I'd weigh without running.

After several false starts, and a few secret relapses, I've quit smoking. I hope. (It was, and remains, one of the most difficult tasks I have ever undertaken.)

If you are a heavy smoker, and you've tried everything

to quit, don't give up hope. One of the great benefits of becoming partially fit is that it eventually leads to a smoke free life. In fact, you'll probably become one of those insufferable born-again non-smokers that puts out those dumb "Thanks-for-not-smoking" signs. Don't ask why it happens, it just does. There's probably some physiological, or at least psychological explanation; no matter, you will have healthy, pink lungs by the time you finish the 5K.

By cutting back on fats and alcohol, my old bottle of Maalox is gathering dust. In fact, there is practically nothing on my medicine shelf now. I don't pay my share of medical costs—though I pay the insurance premiums and the extra taxes caused by people who are not fit.

For the last ten years or more I have felt good, mentally and physically. I mean, really good. Nothing hurts. I look forward to every day, especially if I have time to leash up our lab and take her along for a run. Last year I ran 11 miles in Big Sur, California, walking a couple hills, and thoroughly enjoyed every minute of it. I ran my first marathon on my 50th birthday—slowly, but completely.

Like everyone else, I've had my share of personal and professional setbacks and problems, but through the low times I have always felt physically and mentally sharp. I've experienced sadness and fear, even grief, but I have never gotten discouraged or given up. I don't think I could have handled the difficult times without physical fitness.

I'm completely convinced that there is a direct relationship between self-esteem and health. Without the latter, the former is more difficult. With fitness you feel like anything is possible. Maybe it isn't possible, but you feel like it is.

I feel so good I want everyone to enjoy this sense of well-being. Hence, this book. Believe me, if I can do it, so can you. No matter what shape you're in, or what age.

(This chapter has been approved by my wife, who has a specialty in good sense.)

Don't give up. You'll run the 5K in nine weeks and you'll have your first taste of fitness. Delicious.

☆

Until next week when we take you off the high school track and get you on some trails, Happy Feet!

WEEK NINE

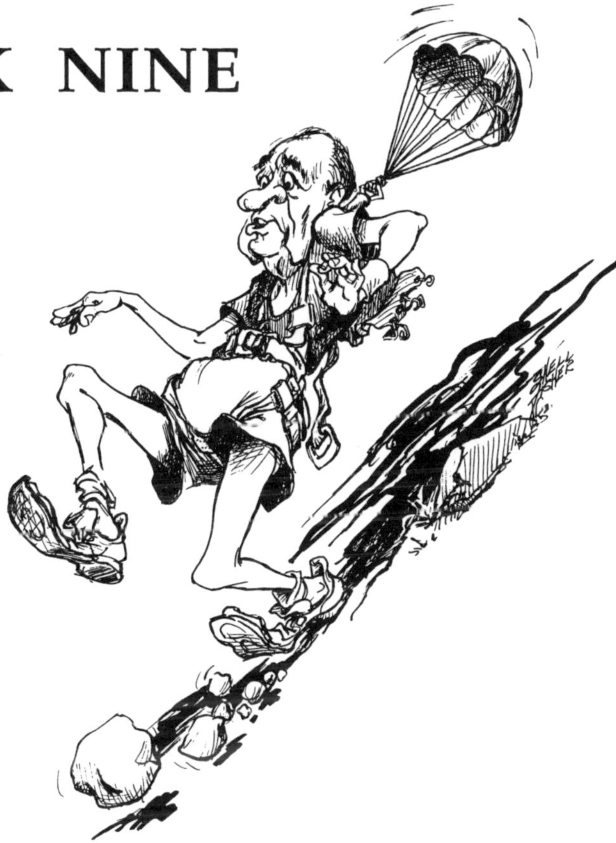

Getting Off Track

YOU FAITHFUL runner(s) have been moving slowly around the high school track and toward your goal of moderate fitness. By now you should have approached the less-than-exalted status of "advanced beginner."

It's time to venture out to the trails and roads, the wide open spaces, paved and unpaved trails.

First, you have to locate them. The best source of information on running in general and where the trails are, is your local running club. Ask a running store or some local runner if there is a club in your community. They are kind of like AA—you don't know they are there until you need them.

Don't feel uncomfortable about approaching a club simply because you are old, overweight, a smoker and in bad shape. There will be others in the club in your condition; you and they are known as new members. Runners, I have found, are an unusual breed of cat: they are tolerant of others, especially beginning runners. They will be glad to map out the trails for you, and recommend lots of choice running areas, both trails and roads.

If you can't find a running club, find some local runners or serious walkers, and ask them to recommend some running trails. Major hotels can give you a "jogging map." Running or sport stores can also help.

You are literally opening new horizons. It's the second best way to see a new city or community, behind only walking. And when you are running you can cover a lot more territory. Note: it's legal and perfectly all right to stop while running just for the purpose of looking at something: a new wildflower or a creative window display. On my first evening in a new city I'll run for about one hour in the downtown area and end up oriented to most of the important sights and landmarks.

Having located the trails, give them a try. You're likely to run into obstacles like roots and rocks, and its okay to slow to a walk and pick your way around. The same applies to hills: don't make yourself run up a hill if it's difficult. Walk, and if you walk briskly, you may keep up your pulse rate and maintain your aerobic workout.

It's a temptation to run fast on the downside of a hill; resist it. That's a good way for beginning runners to get hurt. Just maintain your normal, slow, steady pace.

If you are a music lover, and you like to run by yourself, trails are a wonderful place for a headset. You might as well get as many of your senses involved as possible. If you want to engage your mind, books-on-tape have become increasingly popular. Your local library may have a good selection, and it's free.

☆

Now that we've left the high school track, and graduated to trails, it's time to move on to roads. Next week we'll introduce road running—with the roads' necessary partner: safety.

Until then, Happy Feet! And stop to smell the roses.

WEEK TEN

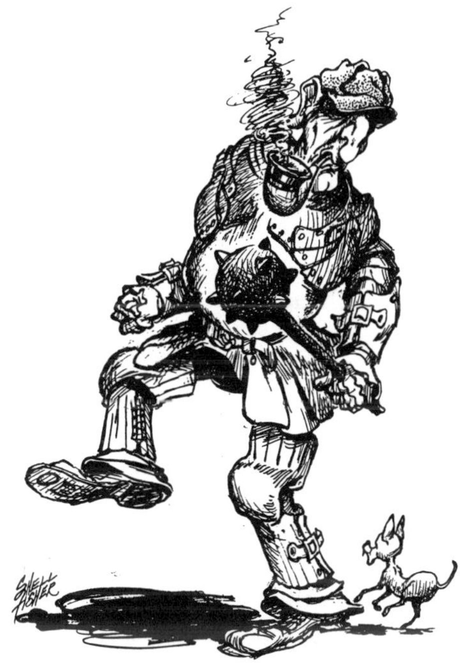

How to Avoid Being an Ugly Road Kill

TIME FOR MORE superficial fitness and training advice. Superficial, to be sure, but irrefutably accurate and undeniably valuable.

Last week we introduced you to trail running. This week we want to talk about roads, but first you need to know about safety.

Contrary to popular opinion, the paved roads are not reserved solely for vehicle traffic. Runners, bikers, skaters, etc., all good tax-payers, have the right to use the road, so long as they do not hinder traffic, and obey traffic laws.

You know that and I know that. Unfortunately, the cars don't know that. Most cars look at runners as trespassers. So you need to protect yourself, to assume that the approaching '67 Buick is out to get you.

There are two good reasons not to get into the path of a car: simple courtesy and the need to remain alive.

Hence, *ve haf rules*:

1. When you share the road with vehicles, run on the left side, facing traffic. If you can, establish eye contact with the driver. That gives you a fraction of a second to respond.

2. If there's a bike path or any sort of trail beside the road, use it. Don't ever run in the roadway if you don't have to. (Another dangling participle that is grammatically permissible.)

3. Never wear dark or neutral clothing, even if you are running in bright sunshine; always wear some major clothing article that is white or yellow. We want drivers to see you.

4. Don't ever wear headphones in traffic; you need all your senses.

5. If you run with companions in traffic, run single file, not side by side. (I saw two mothers running with strollers, side by side on a two lane road. Help!)

6. Never run on high speed roads; that is, any road or highway that has a speed limit in excess of 35 mph. You simply don't have time to react to an inattentive (or hostile!) driver.

7. If you are running downtown in a city, stick to the sidewalks, even if they are crowded. In fact, if you have access to sidewalks in a residential or rural area, use them for safety.

8. Nighttime running can be fun if you have a full moon and an unobstructed surface—but carry a flashlight and flash oncoming drivers. Wearing reflective vests or stripes is best, if you can.

It is surprising how much you can see at night, especially in a neighborhood. There is more light than you would expect. Still, pick up your feet a little higher than normal, to allow for cracks and edges in the roadway.

9. If you run in an area with a lot of dogs, carry an old tennis racquet, or at least a stick.

10. Women runners, regrettably, need special rules. The likelihood of getting attacked is negligible, but you should still adopt a few precautions:

Don't run anywhere by yourself at night. Don't run isolated trails by yourself at anytime of day or night.

Don't run the same route regularly; be unpredictable.

Wear a "Don't mess with me!" attitude. Look like you are alert and in control, and your visible lack of vulnerability should put an attacker off.

If you are attacked, tell him you are HIV positive. If

he doesn't have a weapon, go for his crotch, use your legs, kick hard, and scream your lungs out. Use your voice; scream: "No! No!" to alert others that you need help.

Finally, just use your common sense. Hardly anybody gets hurt running the roads, and the odds are overwhelmingly in your favor. Just acknowledge the risks, and take the necessary steps for your protection.

Now, where do we go? Almost any residential street is nice to run, because you can check out the gardens, homes and the people. At this stage of your training, pick flat neighborhoods or flat country roads. City streets and shopping centers are interesting, so long as you are reasonably prudent. And remember that sightseeing is encouraged.

☆

I think you are ready for a commitment now. Send for the entry form for that 5K race seven weeks from now. Fill it out and send in your entry fee.

Next week we are going to discuss weight changes through running. Until then, Happy Feet! All roads lead to health, if traveled on foot.

WEEK ELEVEN

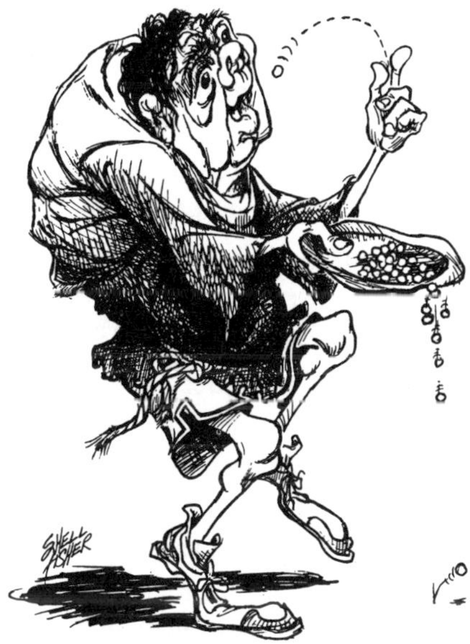

The Final and Ultimate Truth about Weight Loss: Give Peas a Chance

As PROMISED last week, we want to discuss weight control. It's hard to be fit if you are lugging around the equivalent of a few five pound sacks of flour. And extra weight is extra additional pressure on your knees and joints when you run.

I'm the world's foremost authority on weight control. I've gained and lost thousands of pounds, using every conceivable diet—fasting (a Russian diet), grapefruit, chemicals, machines, programs, etc. I've finally discovered the secret to weight control, so listen up! I'm going to save you hundreds of dollars because I've done all the research for you. Here it is.

The only way to lose weight is to burn off more food than you consume, to eat less than your body uses. There is no substitute for this fact. No diet, chemical, machine or program will work unless you reduce the number of calories you eat. If you forked down 100 apples every day, you would gain weight.

Don't despair, however. You can lose weight without too much suffering, too much hunger, by merely reducing the size of the portions of the food you eat. In other words, eat three good, substantial meals a day, but just a little less quantity. Instead of two Fig Newtons with your coffee, have one. Instead of two glasses of wine, have one and a half. Use non-fat dressing for your salad.

It's important that you don't upset your metabolism (don't mess with Mother Nature) by eating too little, or not often enough. Don't skip meals, because your body will just panic and store fat in case you do that again. Eat good, solid meals, with lots of carbos, a little oil and plenty of veggies and salads.

I have a theory, unsubstantiated, that God or somebody assigns everyone a natural weight. If your assigned weight is a good one, and you can gorge without gaining, you're lucky. If you are like me and most people, your natural weight is too high, and you have to struggle to keep it down.

Suppose your weight is about 20 pounds too much. You probably take in about 2,500 calories a day to maintain that weight. (Unless you are a small person, then it's less.)

All you need to do to lose weight, then, is to eat about 2,000 calories a day.

So, buy a book that gives a caloric measure for all foods, and a small food scale. Figure out the total calories of your normal day, then cut that about 15 to 20 percent. You don't want to lose too much, too fast, because it discombobulates your metabolism. Any more than that will trigger a starvation panic in your body. All responsible authorities on nutrition agree that a pound or two a week is plenty. And you need nutrients; don't get your calories primarily from potato chips and beer.

About every February I lose eight pounds (holiday excesses) in six weeks. Here is a typical day's consumption:

Breakfast:	2 cups cooked oatmeal and bran (250 calories),1 banana (100), coffee (5), 1 tsp. sugar (15)
Morning Snack:	1 cup popcorn made with oil (40)
Lunch:	1.2 oz. instant soup (150), 6 oz. sunflower seeds in shell (65) 2½ inch chocolate chip cookie (55) 4 oz. red wine (100)
Afternoon Snack:	1 cup popcorn made with oil (40), coffee with sugar (20)
Evening:	1½ oz. whiskey (100), 1 cup egg noodles (100), 1 cup low-fat

yogurt (145), ¼ cup romano cheese (180) and seasonings for sauce; 1 cup broccoli (50), with 2 Tbs. non-fat dressing (30), 6 oz. red wine (250), coffee (20) and one Fig Newton (55).

That's a total of 1,825 calories and the fat intake was way under the recommended 30 percent of total calorie intake.

IMPORTANT! To lose weight, you really do have to measure, weigh and write down your calories. It's too easy to forget that Ritz cracker you ate at a friend's desk.

When I put this menu in my fitness column in the newspaper, there was shocked reaction that I included whiskey and wine on a diet. It was intentional, I assure you. I want readers to know that anything is okay in moderation, as long as you are getting proper nutrition. The key is the total number of calories consumed. Sixty-five percent of the public drinks alcohol; they can become fit and lose weight without giving it up. Also, there is considerable research that alcohol in moderation (one or two glasses of wine a day), particularly red wine, has health benefits. This book, as you can see, is not a program of deprivation.

Eating as described, I was seldom hungry or uncomfortable, and I had a couple-three lapses, when we went out or traveled. But since my six foot body uses about 2,200 calories a day to maintain my weight, the pounds and inches slowly dropped off when I reduced my caloric intake to about 1,800. I'm still about 10 pounds overweight, but I can live with that.

Many of the concepts in this chapter are taken from the sixteen week "Weigh of Life" course offered at the Community Hospital of Monterey Peninsula, California. My wife had the good sense and dedication to take the course, and I stole the ideas from her. And they work.

☆

Next week we will discuss the effect of exercise on weight loss. Until then, Happy Feet! Remember that light foods give you a light step.

WEEK TWELVE

I just chow'd down 2 ½ miles worth of potato chips.

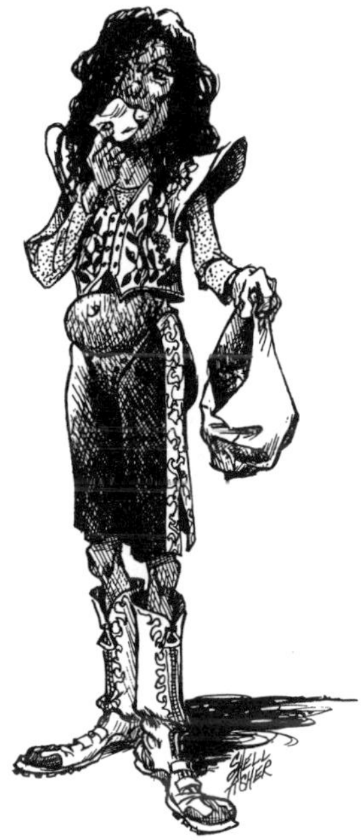

Eight 2½ Inch Chocolate Chip Cookies, Free!

How are you doing? For those who started with us, you have been training now about three months. Have you had a pleasant run yet?

Possibly, but not likely. As I recall, when I started it was more than three months before I had an enjoyable run, and then it was only a couple of miles.

Let's review where you should be at this stage of training for the 5K you have chosen to run.

You should be running for a continuous 20 minutes, either on a track or trails or roads, in good quality running shoes, with an elevated pulse rate of 130 to 150 beats per minute, three times a week. (Remember, for your exercise pulse rate, subtract your age from 220, then take 70 percent of that.)

If you are doing more than that, it's good training for the 5K, it's good for your weight and muscle tone, but you get a strong, healthy heart with the minimum training: 20 minutes, three times a week.

If your training is walking, you should be at a brisk (15 minute mile) pace for at least 45 minutes a day, at least three times a week.

Hopefully, you have reduced your fat intake to less than 30 percent of your total calories, and you are avoiding saturated fats (animal and dairy products) as much as possible. And you are taking advantage of the numerous low fat, and especially, non-fat products on the market.

Your consumption of complex carbohydrates—potatoes, pastas, breads—should have increased to make up for your reduced red meat intake. If you have done all this, you probably feel much better already.

You should not have had any injuries, because your training is so basic, and presumably you have learned to live with a few niggling discomforts and aches.

This week we want to continue our discussion of weight control and exercise. Perhaps "weight" isn't the proper word; "size" may be more appropriate. If you don't intentionally diet, running will change the size of your waist, hips, thighs, etc. Pounds will move around, even if your weight doesn't change.

The use of muscles makes them larger and denser—and heavier. If you are training well and not losing weight, it's most likely because the fat around your hips or waist or thighs is now heavier muscle in your legs.

But if you want to lose weight, exercise is a terrific way to supplement reduction in the calories you consume. You burn up about 70 to 80 calories an hour watching TV. You burn about 100 calories for every mile you run (or walk, or sprint). So if you run three miles in 30 minutes, you will use about 300 calories in one half hour. Or about 600 calories if you run for an hour—520 more than watching TV. That's eight 2½ inch chocolate chip cookies! And you come out even!

Now here's the best part: We all have a little furnace built into our body—I think it is in the left shoulder—called metabolism. It burns up those calories that, in excess, cause so much mischief. (And grief!) Exercise stokes the furnace so that it keeps burning long after you quit your workout! Another miracle! I think it's nature's way of rewarding you for being good.

If you combine exercise with a diet, you can eat more and still lose weight, because you are burning up the food that you are eating faster than normal. So if you need an incentive to make one more mile, think of it as 10 to 15 pistachios or a cold beer.

In last week's chapter, I mentioned that in a typical day of dieting I will consume about 1,900 calories. If I throw in a four mile run, then my body has only 1,500 calories, much less than it uses. End result: weight loss . . . clothes start to fit again . . . big meal at the local Rib BBQ neatly rationalized.

Remember when I asked you to get your cholesterol and vital signs recorded about six weeks ago? Okay, so you've put it off. But it's not too late. Your bad cholesterol, your blood pressure and your pulse rate are all going down—and your good cholesterol is going up. This is all good for your ego, your good humor and your longevity.

(The advice in this chapter has been approved, believe it or not, by nutritionists at Community Hospital of the Monterey Peninsula.)

☆

Next week is a subject so abhorrent, so distasteful, that I won't even tell you about it. If I did, you would never return to this book. All your fitness work would be wasted. Trust me, come back next week, and, until then, Happy Feet! And eat your salads.

WEEK THIRTEEN

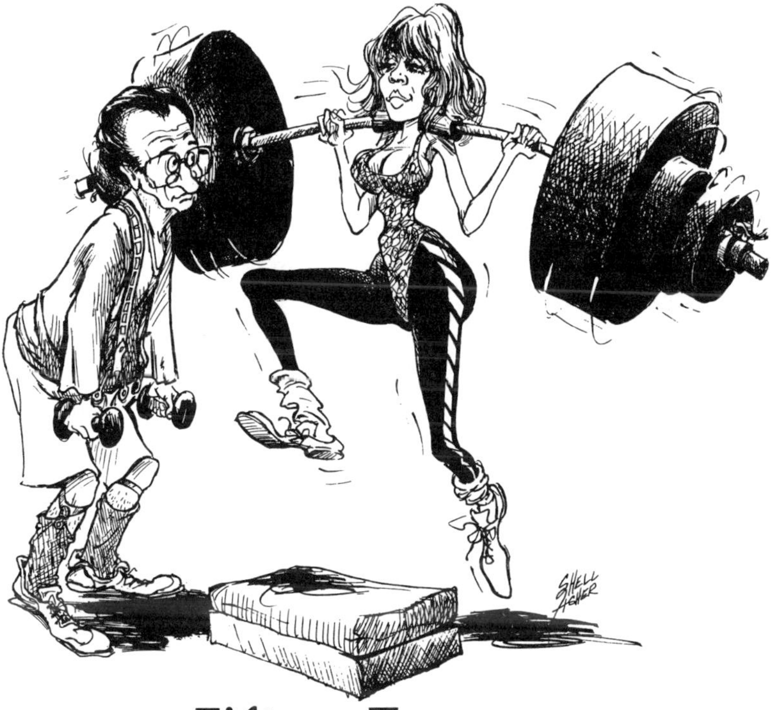

Fifteen Tons and What Do You Get . . . .

A BOOK THAT gives advice on fitness, even semi-fitness, would not be complete without a discussion of resistance training. That is a euphemism for weight lifting.

Stop! Don't leave! I know you have no interest whatsoever in lifting barbells, but bear with me for at least a few paragraphs. You'll be glad you did.

Looking in the mirror at age 40 got me started in running and at least partial fitness. A swimming pool got me started with resistance training.

A couple of years ago I went swimming for the first time in 20 years and found I couldn't make a lap without my arms and shoulders tiring. So, I thought I'd try moving weights around and see what happened.

A professional showed me how to work the Nautilus-type machines in a health club, and I'm here to tell you that it is not as bad as you would think. In fact, there are some good points to weight training:

1. *Bullies won't kick sand in your face anymore.*
2. *If you are over 40, it gives you something to look at in the mirror besides liver spots.*

It's only been a couple of years, and I am getting round places that used to be flat, and flat places that used to be lumpy. I suppose everybody thinks I'm on steroids. I found a neat new muscle behind the top of my arms, about the shape of a banana slug, and I stand in front of the mirror and twist my arms to check it out. (I'm convinced that if mirrors had not been invented, there would be no bodybuilding industry.)

3. *Believe it not, working out with those machines actually feels good.*

I know what you are saying: Burleigh has lost it. But you should try it sometime. If you don't do physical work for a living, you can get a sensual pleasure from the effort involved.

I don't care for free weights—barbells—but the machines in the health clubs have been developed to work certain muscles, and you can control exactly how much effort you want to expend, and in what manner. My trainer had me do 15 repetitions of each machine twice, three times a week. And the goal is to set the weight level so that your muscle is exhausted by the time you reach 15. You end up with a nice, heavy, relaxed feeling in your arms and shoulders.

The trainer told me that I would improve with time, and increase the level of my weights, but it hasn't worked out that way. I'm moving the same pounds I did two years ago. I guess my body is deteriorating at the same speed that I'm building it up.

4. *It doesn't take much time.*

The experts say you need to let your muscles recover for a day after a workout, and recommend that you only have three sessions a week. Most people can do all the repetitions they need, on all the machines they need, in less than 45 minutes. I only do about 25 minutes, unhurriedly, and it seems to maintain my little bulges. Muscle bulges.

5. *Quite often the scenery in health clubs is spectacular. Enough said.*

There is one downside to resistance training:

Membership in a health club for a single can be $30 to $60 a month. You can buy free weights (yuk) for a couple hundred dollars, or you can purchase a home gym similar to the Nautilus machines for around $2,000. I suppose it's cheaper than tennis, golf, skiing and polo, but it's a lot more expensive than running.

Well, time to go oil up my body and stand in front of the mirror.

(The advice in this chapter has not been approved by anyone even remotely connected with weight training.)

☆

Next week we discuss, among other things, that always provocative and stimulating subject of liquids and exercise.

Until then, Happy Biceps! And eat your peaches.

WEEK FOURTEEN

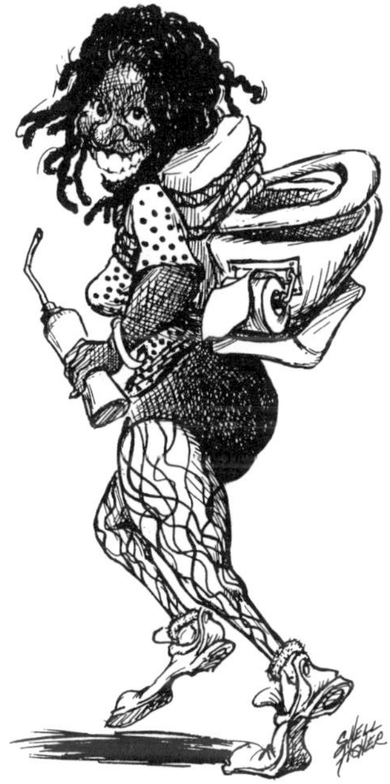

If You Drown, You've Had Too Much Water

Now, on to our subject for the week: liquids and exercise.

About all you have to know about water and long distance running is that you have to drink water (hydrate!) the day before, the night before and during the event, to the point where it's seeping out your ears.

Well, perhaps that's a slight exaggeration. But we cannot emphasize too much how important water is when you exercise. All kinds of bad things happen when you dehydrate.

I know whereof I speak. One of the worst experiences of my life occurred during a 22 mile training run for my first marathon. I think it was 22 miles; my mind went, along with the rest of my body. I could hardly find the car and my wife had to drive me home, and I spent several hours close to convulsions. All of it unnecessary. All because I didn't take enough water.

If you can see color in your urine before a long run, you're in trouble. It should be clear. You need a lot more water before the run. The only way to drink too much water is if you drown.

As you know, when you exercise you get hot, and to cool off nature makes you sweat. But you need to maintain 60 percent of your total body weight (70 percent of muscles) in water. If you lose too much water in sweat (dehydrate), you cannot perform physically, and you risk injury to your kidneys.

Common symptoms are chills, clammy skin, throbbing heartbeat and nausea. Later and more serious stages are hallucinations, deafness, visual problems and swollen tongue.

Have we gotten your attention?

You know how it is when you go for a walk in the Sahara, take a wrong turn and end up surrounded by hundreds of miles of sand? We've all had that experience, and it makes you realize water is more important to you than food—at least in terms of sustaining life. You can do without food, completely, for a couple of weeks, but without water you would expire in a few days.

Dr. Donald S. Robertson of the Providence medical center PRISM wrote an article titled "Are You Drinking Enough Water?"

I've been reading about running and fitness, including the importance of water, for 20 years, and I still learned some new information from Dr. Robertson. Particularly concerning weight control.

Did you know that a decrease in water intake will cause fat deposits to increase while an increase in water consumption can actually reduce deposits?

Here's why: one of the liver's prime functions is to metabolize stored fat into usable energy for the body. If you don't drink enough water, your kidneys don't function properly. When they don't, some of their workload is dumped onto the liver—distracting it from its main function of burning fat.

If you divert the liver's attention to other chores, it metabolizes less fat, so more fat remains stored in the the body, and weight loss stops.

It follows, then, that if you drink the proper amount of water, your kidneys will operate normally. The liver, not being called upon to help one of it organ colleagues, will go about its function of metabolizing that mayonnaise and butter sauce you had last week.

It's amazing what happens after you drink a glass of water. All kinds of great things go on. I try to remember to drink a cup of water every time I have a cup of coffee, and a glass of water several times a day. I try hard.

Almost everything that happens inside your body involves water, according to *Prevention Magazine*'s book, "Food and Nutrition." It helps digest your oatmeal breakfast (with fruit, etc.!) and carries the dissolved nutrients to each cell in your body. It's like a subway system, albeit a small one. A miracle!

Water is a thermostat, except it keeps you at 98.6° F instead of the outside 70° F. Sweat, you know!

Remember how the Tin Man in "The Wizard of Oz." rusted and froze up? That would happen to you if you didn't have water to lubricate your joints.

There is no strict formula for how much water you need—some doctors say 8 ounces, eight times a day. An average non-active adult, according to Leroy Perry, President of the International Sportsmedicine Institute of Los Angeles, should drink a half-ounce of water per day for every pound of bodyweight. That's a lot of water—10 eight ounce glasses a day for a 160 pound person—but you won't drown. Sorry, coffee and booze don't count. Both can be diuretics.

I wish I had enough space to describe in detail how water flushes out bacteria, dead cells, sewage, decomposing mice and rancid brussels sprouts, but I have to move on. Suffice it to say that water does a body good.

As a practical matter, you don't need too much liquid to complete a 5K, but as you get around five to 10 miles, or 45 to 60 minutes of exertion, you need to keep the water level protected.

Watch the pros. Jimmy Connors will drink a gallon of water the day before a match. Top marathoners, such as Brad Hawthorne, carry a water bottle with them all day before the race.

Finally it has recently been discovered that water increases the ability of your muscles to store glycogen (carbohydrate), that wonderful stuff that lets you run forever.

(Many thanks to the Nutrition Department of the Community Hospital of the Monterey Peninsula.)

☆

Eat your broccoli, get your pulse rate up, and, until next week, Happy Feet!

WEEK FIFTEEN

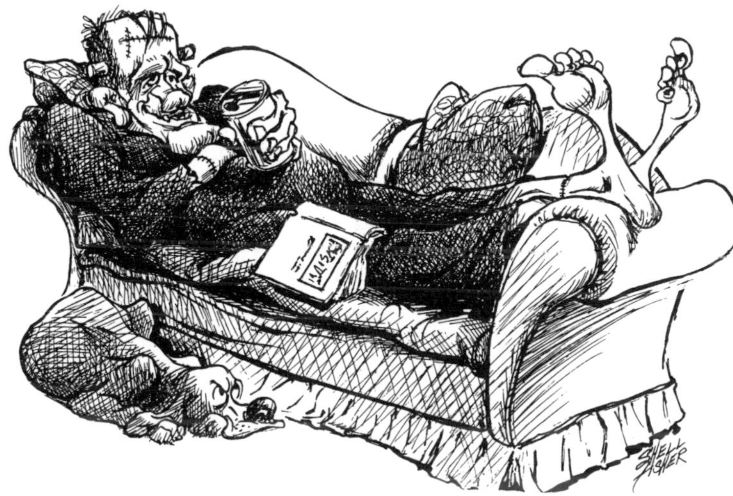

The Devil Made Me Stay at Home

I PRETTY MUCH follow the advice I've been giving you in this book. Actually, I get so much sensual pleasure from running now that I'll put in three to five miles whenever the opportunity presents itself, such as good weather, a holiday or a vacation.

Now, with that in mind, here's what I did recently. I got home from work on a beautiful evening, the dog was jumping around in anticipation of a run on the beach, the tide was out and it looked like a beautiful sunset coming up. It was time to change and drive to the ocean.

So I said to hell with it, popped a beer, apologized to the dog, plugged in a Peter Gabriel tape and stretched out to finish the last few chapters of a trashy spy novel. The run would be undone.

And did I feel guilty? Of course. That's one of the hazards of being a runner. You know it's good for you and that you'll feel better when you finish your run, and you might even have one of those great runs that are so exhilarating you don't want to stop. But I still occasionally just don't do it. Shine it on.

The point is, of course, that you don't have to be a fanatic about running. Or fitness, or eating properly. No harm is done if you skip a day or a week of running or go crazy in the ice cream store. Frankly, I'm suspicious of the person who treats this sport like a religion, never faltering or backsliding.

Sometimes you miss a lot of runs involuntarily, because of injury. And you'll still feel guilty. I go for a run when I have a cold or minor illness, but I'll stay home if I have a fever.

You'll find, however, that as you become fit you won't get sick as much. I had my first cold in three years a couple of months ago. Running also strengthened the muscles in my back, and I haven't needed to go to a chiropractor for about ten years.

Finally, if you are choosing to take a vacation from running, keep in mind that after a few weeks you lose your conditioning, and it's like starting all over again.

Now, having told you it's okay to just simply flake out occasionally, for no reason at all, I want to address the runner who flakes out too much.

There are lots of excuses for not running, and none of them are any good; none are acceptable.

The most common is lack of time. Sorry, that doesn't sell. All you are saying is that you put running on a priority scale below that of everything else you are doing. You are saying that running isn't important. You are putting the pursuit of the dollar, or a social event, or even a TV show, ahead of good health. Perhaps you are saying that you, yourself, are not important.

I beg to differ; if you are a veteran runner, you know how important it is to your health and well being. You know it is a major source of energy. You know the impact that it has on your cholesterol, blood pressure, pulse rate and weight.

If you are a beginning runner, you can't appreciate the value of running until you've done it for a couple of years. But that is still no excuse. Everybody has to do things they don't want to do, so keep at it, rookie, until you appreciate it.

Another popular excuse for not hitting the roads is that you are tired. Hard day's work, bad night's sleep, whatever. That doesn't do it, either. In fact, you know in your heart that if you drag yourself out for a few miles you will feel much better for the rest of the day. Cobwebs disappear. Spirits rejuvenate.

Some folks, particularly beginning runners, use injury, past or present, as an excuse. Quite often it is a legitimate reason to stay home, but often it is merely a reluctance to make the effort.

It's a mind-set. If you decide you are going to run, no matter what, you will. You can make the time if you want to, you can give the run priority, and as the ad says, *just do it.*

We all want to feel good and live a long time. Everybody. I've heard people say they don't want to live through the infirmities of old age—loss of hearing and sight, incontinence, memory loss, etc.—but when the chips are down, they choose life over death.

It's the life force, and there are very, very few exceptions.

With that in mind, I have to tell you that the goal of longevity and good health is available to you. Regrettably, it is not yet in pill form. It carries the labels of exercise and good nutrition, both of which can be unpleasant to some folks.

Some people, those who are intellectually oriented as opposed to the sensual, may never enjoy exercise. But that doesn't mean that they do not have to exercise. They still have to do the bare minimum for a healthy heart, lowered cholesterol and blood pressure and stronger bones. That amounts to about 20 minutes of aerobic activity, three times a week.

The fact that it is disagreeable is no excuse. We all have to do things we don't want to do.

Every job, every profession, is occasionally unpleasant, tedious, boring, and repetitive.

You think movie stars have it easy? They often get up at 4 a.m. for makeup, spend hours and hours memorizing lines, then film the same scene over and over and over again.

Have you ever watched a lawyer's or doctor's eyes glaze over while you're telling him your problems?

As a judge, I have one of the most interesting jobs in the world—always changing, often amusing and usually stimulating. But I have to advise individuals of their constitutional rights a zillion times a day, and it's numbing.

I challenge you to name any job that isn't disagreeable upon occasion.

Having established that we all must do things we don't want to do in order to make a living, why don't we do the same thing to make a better and longer life?

All it amounts to is that magic 20 minutes three times a week and eating more nutritional food while pushing away the delicious bad stuff. (And, of course, no smoking.)

There are only two valid excuses for not becoming at least half-fit: physical disability and lack of will power. There is nothing that anybody can do to alleviate these conditions. (My wife disagrees. She says that if you improve your self-perception, and come to value yourself, you will gain will power.)

Assuming you are not disabled and have a moderate amount of willpower, there is no question that you will feel better and live longer if you are at least semi-fit.

So, go for it. NO EXCUSES. NO BOZOS.

☆

Next week is your first race, perhaps your first athletic feat. Makes you nervous, doesn't it? It's normal to be snarly; if your spouse doesn't understand, show him or her this book. Next week you will have an experience that you will never forget.

Hang in there, eat your bananas, and until next week, Happy Feet!

THE LAST WEEK

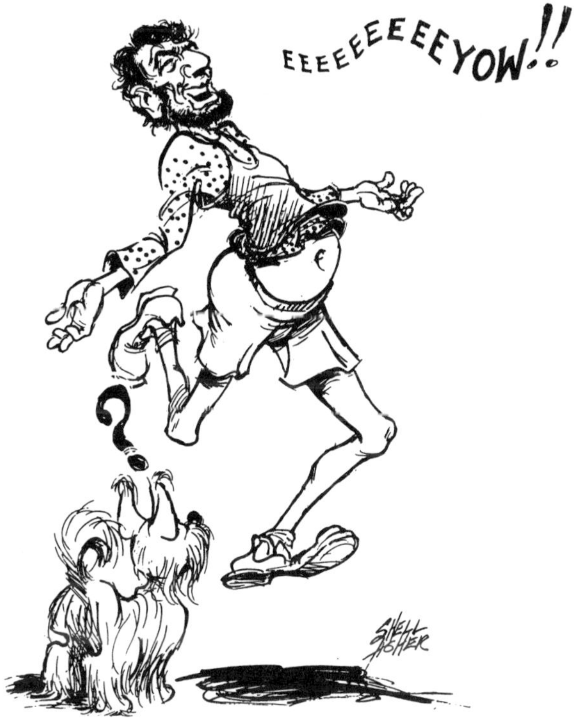

When Are the Olympic Trials?

I CAN TELL what mood you are in right now, depending on the time of day.

If you are reading this before your 5K race, you are nervous, uptight and irritable. You slept poorly last night, and you are asking yourself, why am I doing this?

I know how you feel. I was a basket case for my first footrace. I wasn't sure I could finish. I wasn't even sure I would survive! It was the most active and strenuous thing I had done in 25 years and I was scared.

If you are reading this after the race, you are a different person. You know you can run more than three miles and you feel terrific. All the suffering was worth it; all the hours spent running down the roads paid off. A 5K piece of cake. Gimme a 10K.

You really are a different person than you were when you started training four months ago. Your pulse rate is lower—so your heart is not working so hard—and your blood pressure is probably lower than it's been in years.

Your bad cholesterol is at least 10 percent lower than before, and your good cholesterol is higher. Your bones are stronger, and you've strengthened the muscles in your back and legs.

Most of the changes in your body are not visible; what can be seen, though, is your new confidence, your new pride in your physical condition.

When you see your aunt for the first time in a year, she won't notice the new you until she's been around long enough to sense the change in your personality.

And that, dear readers, is why I wrote this book—to increase the level of fitness in your community. My goal is ambitious but easily stated: I want to have more fit people in your community.

The 5K is the perfect vehicle for fitness. You simply can't run 3.1 miles without getting your body into shape. You can't turn off the TV, walk outside and run a 5K without a lot of training. And you did it!

When I started writing this book, I said I was going to tell you how to train to run a 5K, and that if you did what I told you, you would end up semi-fit. Well, I lied.

If you ran the 5K today, without stopping and walking, you are 100 percent fit. Congratulations!

Now, here is my hidden agenda: I hope you have caught the bug, that today is just a beginning, a starting point for you. I hope that you will continue your training for the sheer joy of it, regardless of any physical or mental goals.

You will, of course, miss a few days or even weeks of running, but the great majority of those who finish the 5K today will continue with good health and good feelings.

May we suggest a new goal for you: train for a 10K. Give yourself about six months to gradually increase your distance and time to handle 6.2 miles. Let's hope that in a few years you will be like most long time runners—you'll have so many race shirts you won't have a place to store them all! And one of them should say:

FORMER ROAD SLUG.
Now, Supercilious, Holier-than-thou, Patronizing,
Pretentious, Overbearing, Intolerant,
Condescending RUNNER!

☆

Happy Feet! And eat your chocolate mocha fudge ice cream. Nobody's perfect.

EGO TRIP PAGE

	Road Slug Statistics (Start of Program)	Semi-Fit Statistics (End of Program)
Blood Pressure		
Pulse Rate (Resting)		
Weight		
Good Cholesterol		
Bad Cholesterol		
Lipids		
Waist (Inches)		
Thigh (Inches)		
Calf (Inches)		
Comments:		